PERRY'S SECRET

MW00761954

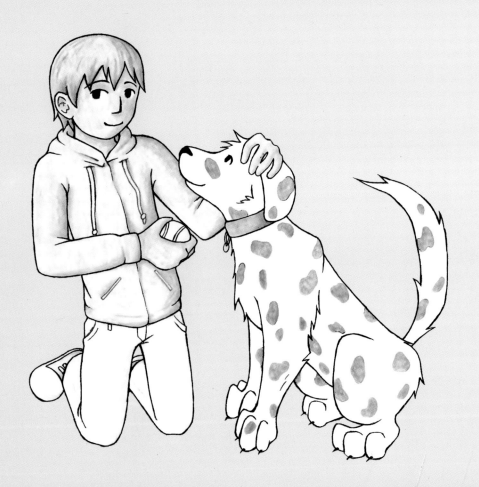

"For Perry"

ISBN 978-0-9842147-9-2

Perry's Secret Copyright 2013 by Jill Roberson-Blatt

Illustrated by Alyssa Guy

Designed and Printed by Panacea Press - Murfreesboro, Tennessee

All rights reserved, no part of this publication may be reproduced, transmitted
in any form by any means, electronic, mechanical, photocopy, recording
or otherwise, without written permission from the publisher, except as
provided by USA copyright law.

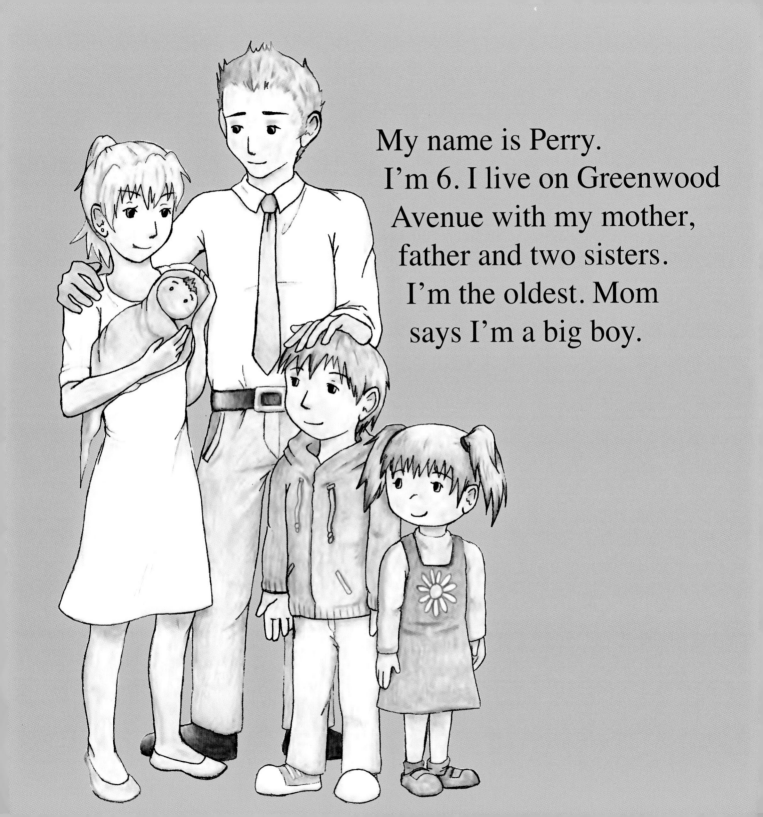

My name is Perry.
I'm 6. I live on Greenwood
Avenue with my mother,
father and two sisters.
I'm the oldest. Mom
says I'm a big boy.

Mrs. Ash is my 1st grade teacher.
She wears ruby red lipstick and smells like cotton.
The best time of day is Art when we can make
projects to hang on the wall. I like recess too.
Tag is my favorite.

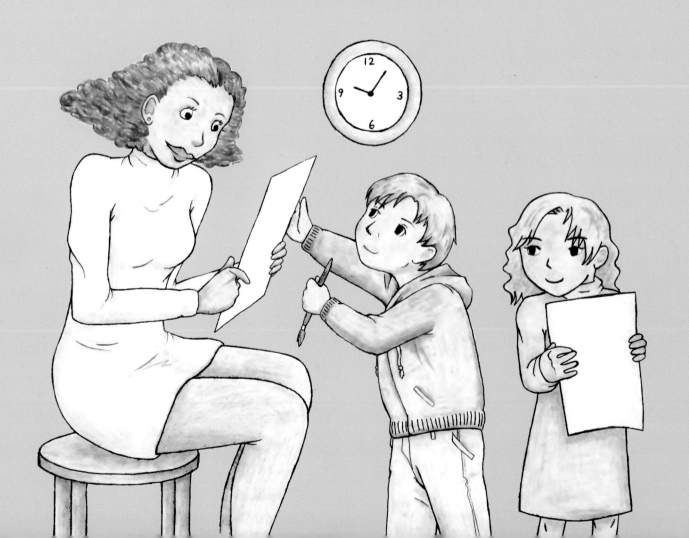

After school at home Mom fixes me my favorite snack. Milk and graham crackers. Yummy.

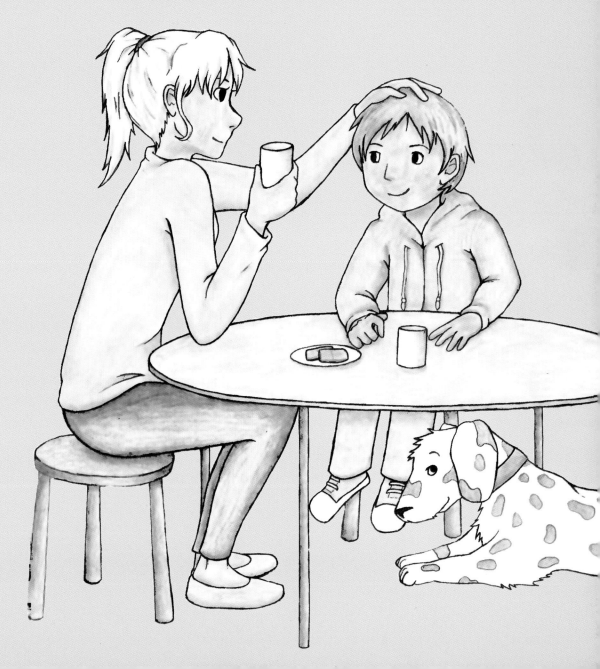

Today Mom said she had a big surprise. Boy do I love surprises. She said my uncle was coming to visit and would be staying with us for a couple of days. She said we would all have a lot of fun and maybe even get to go swimming. But only if it doesn't rain.

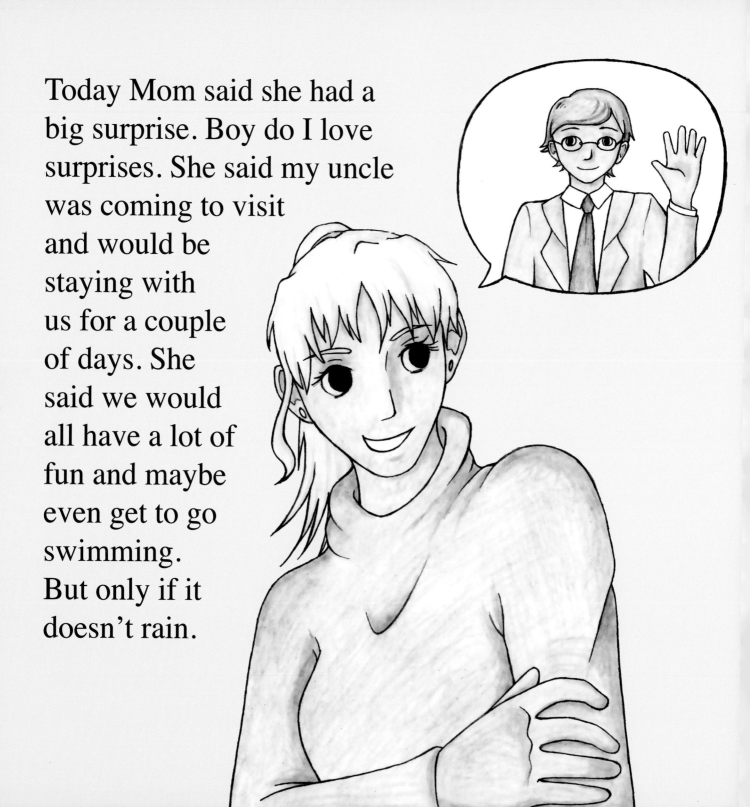

I don't really remember my Uncle Jim. Mom says his work is very important and he works for a very big company. Mom says he travels all the time and has been all over the world. I can't wait to ask him all about his adventures. I was so excited for him to come I couldn't finish my snack.

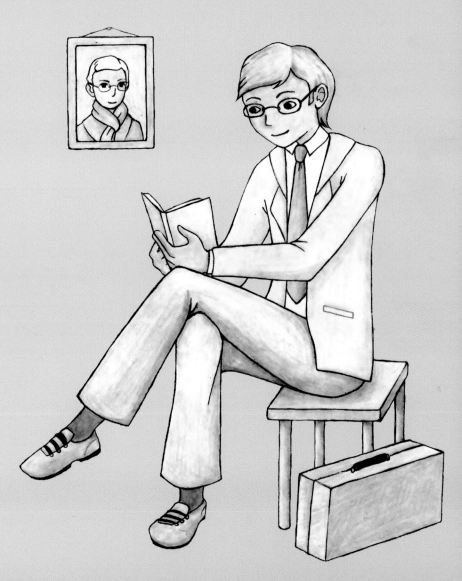

The day my Uncle Jim was to come I was so excited I could hardly sit still. Mrs. Ash had to tell me twice to stop squirming and wiggling. I couldn't wait for the dismissal bell to ring and go home and hear about all of Uncle Jim's adventures.

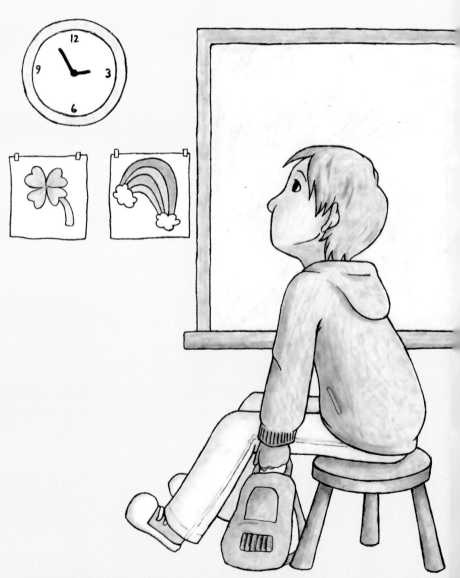

When I got home Uncle Jim was sitting at the kitchen table drinking coffee with Mom. He came over and gave me a big hug. While Mom fixed my snack I sat and listened and asked Uncle Jim a million questions about everywhere he has been. We talked and talked until Dad came home and Mom said "Dinnertime."

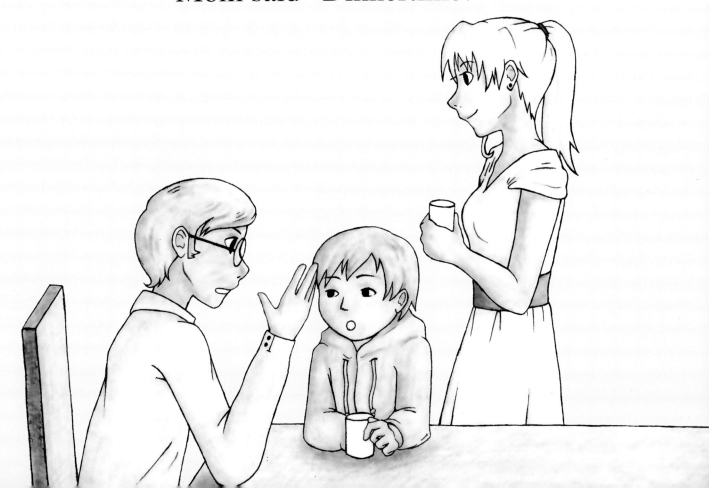

After supper we all gathered in the den to watch TV and do some more catching up. Uncle Jim asked if I wanted to sit in his lap while he told more stories about his travels. He helped me up and I sat big and tall. My sisters are too little to do that. They are just babies.

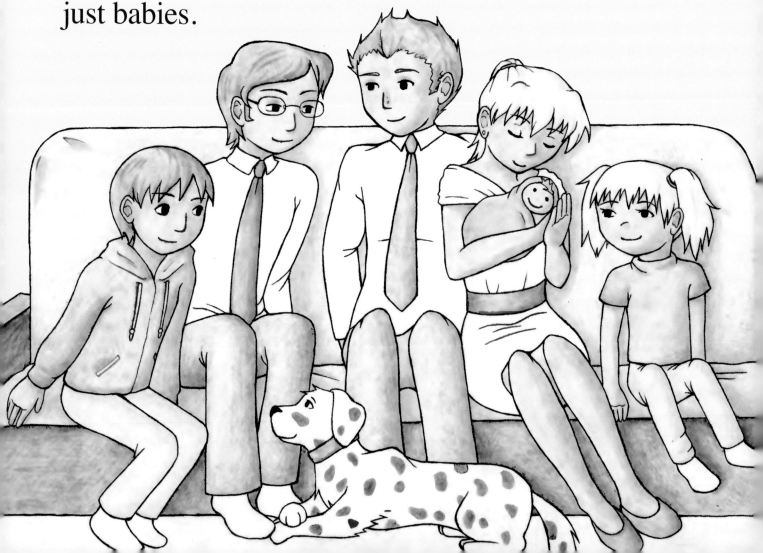

Then Mom said it was getting late and it's time for bed. I hopped off Uncle Jim's lap and Dad helped me brush my teeth. "Uncle Jim will be sleeping in your room in the spare bed," I groaned.
Dad pinkie swore he wouldn't snore.

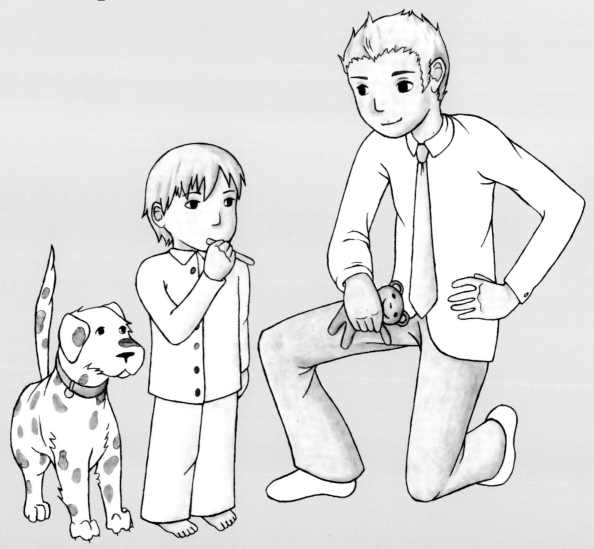

That night around 9 o'clock I heard Uncle Jim come into my room and start to unpack his suitcase and brush his teeth. I could tell he was trying to be quiet but I heard a muffled "ouch" as he tripped over some of my toys.

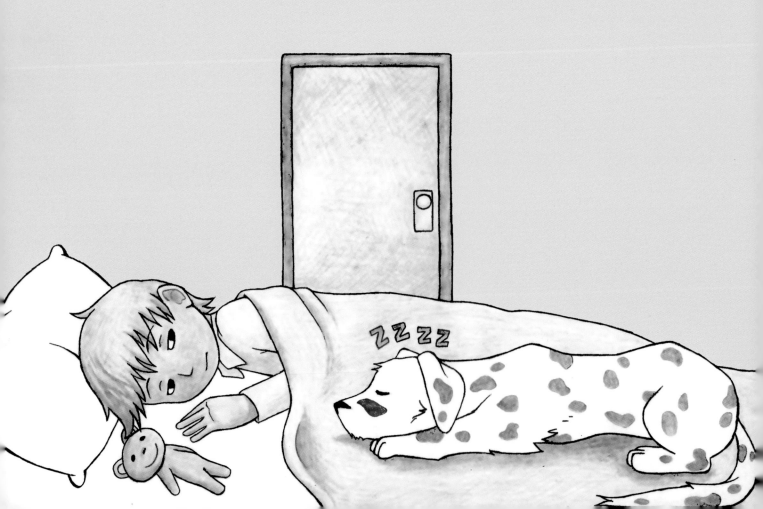

I wasn't fully awake but I wasn't sleeping when Uncle Jim came to my bed. He was whispering for me to keep my eyes closed and stay quiet. I felt something under the covers go where Mom said nobody should go. It only lasted a few minutes but it felt like forever. Was I dreaming?

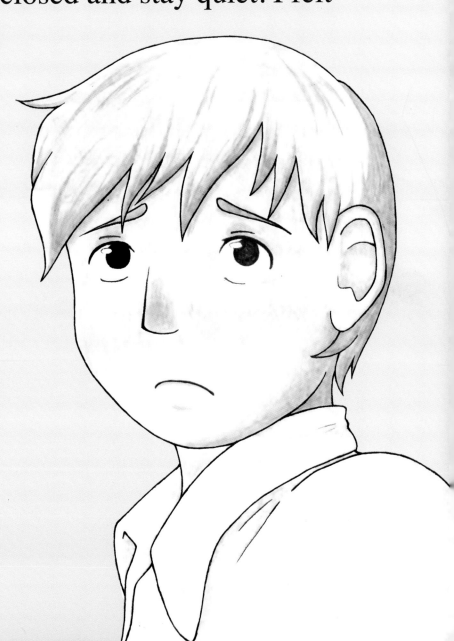

When it was over, I heard
Uncle Jim get into bed and
fall asleep. I couldn't sleep. I
was wide awake in case Uncle
Jim woke up and tried to do
that again. I didn't know what
I should do. Should I tell my
Mom and Dad? Should
I yell for help? Why
didn't I stop him?

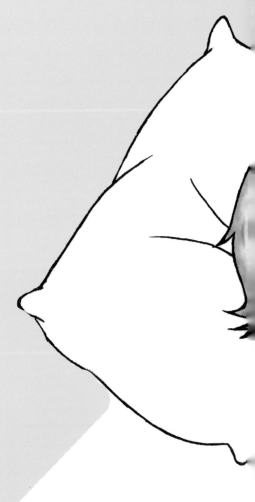

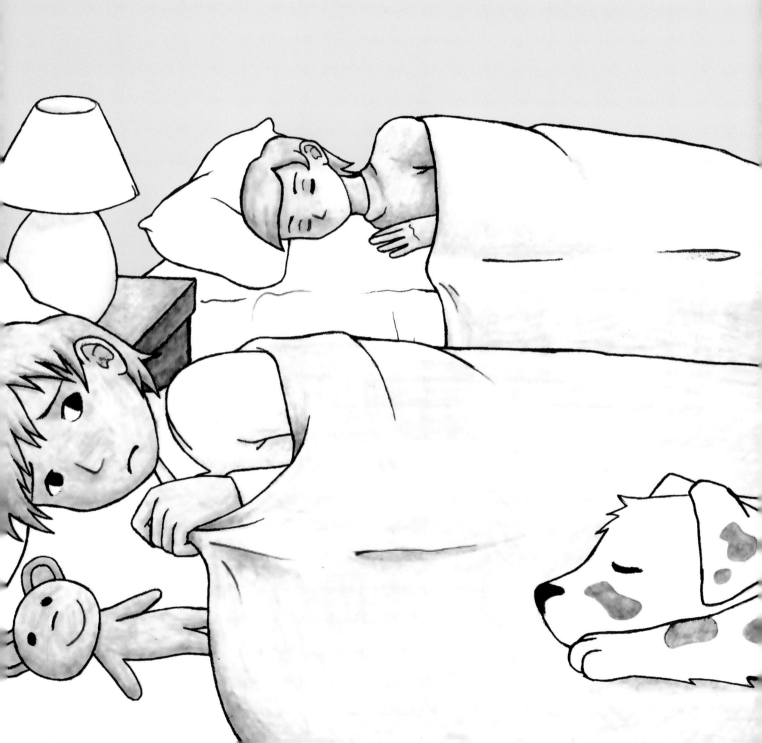

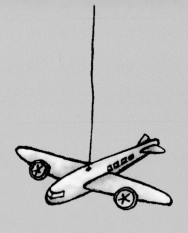

The next day was Saturday.
I didn't wake up until
Uncle Jim had left the room.
I couldn't remember
everything that happened
but that I felt very bad inside.
My stomach began to
hurt and big alligator tears
began to fall on my pillow.

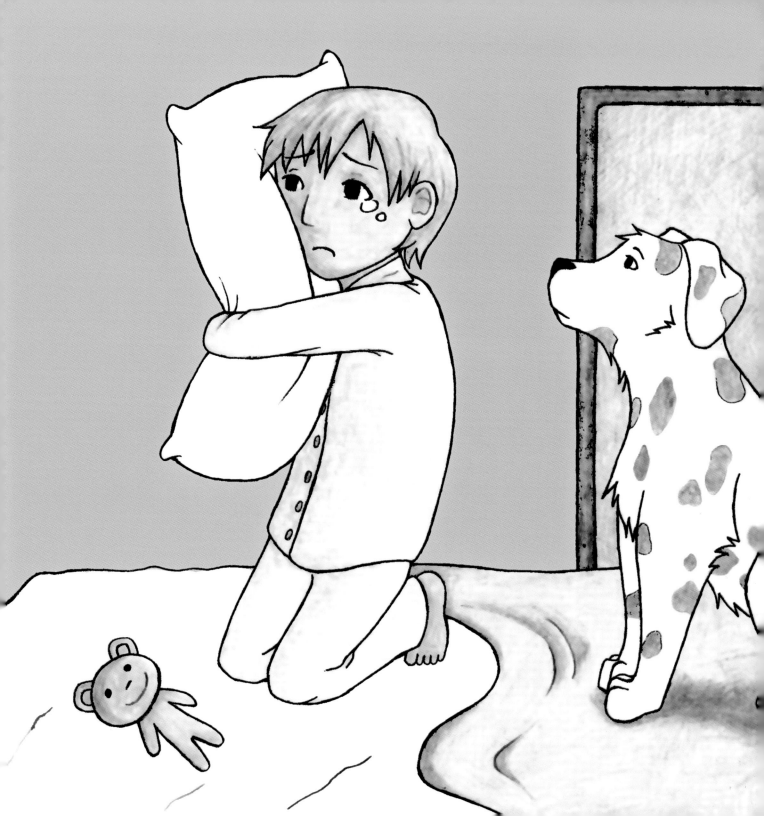

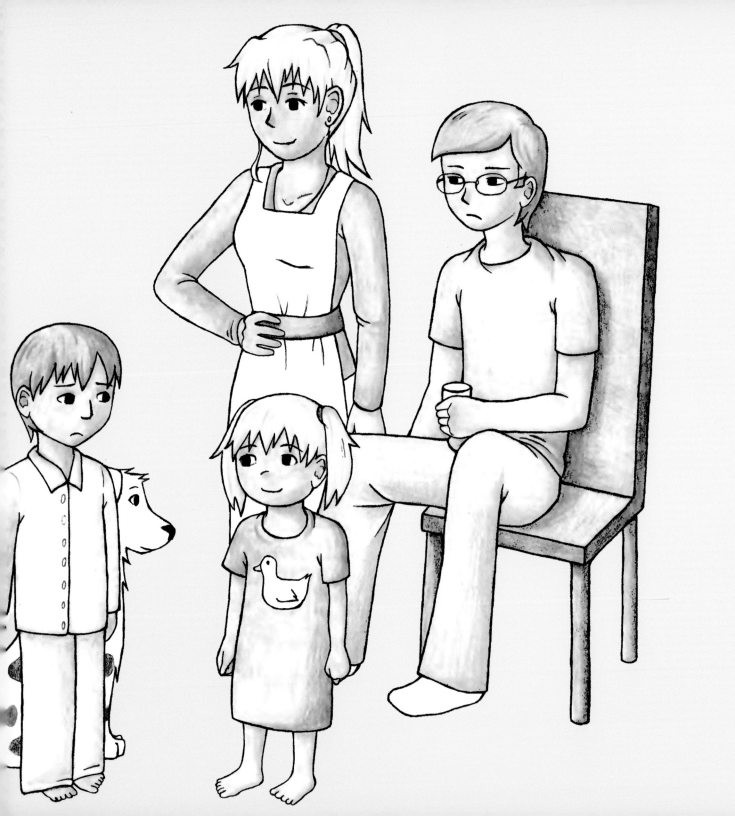

I finally got out of bed and went into the kitchen where Mom was making pancakes. Uncle Jim was sitting at the table drinking coffee. "Did you sleep well?" he asked. I remained quiet. Mom asked if anything was wrong. "I don't feel good," I told her and asked if I could go back to bed.

"You don't want pancakes? But they are your favorite!" I couldn't eat any breakfast. I didn't know what I should do. Should I tell my mother? What if I got in trouble? What if she didn't believe me? I left the kitchen without permission and went back to my room. I laid back down and curled into a small ball trying my best to disappear.

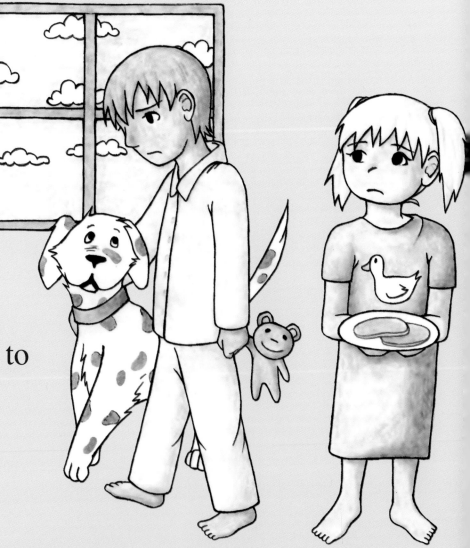

Nighttime came and Uncle Jim came to my bed again. "You're not going to tell anyone about our little secret are you Perry?" I held my breath but I wanted to scream. This went on for 2 more nights until finally Uncle Jim said it was time for him to leave.

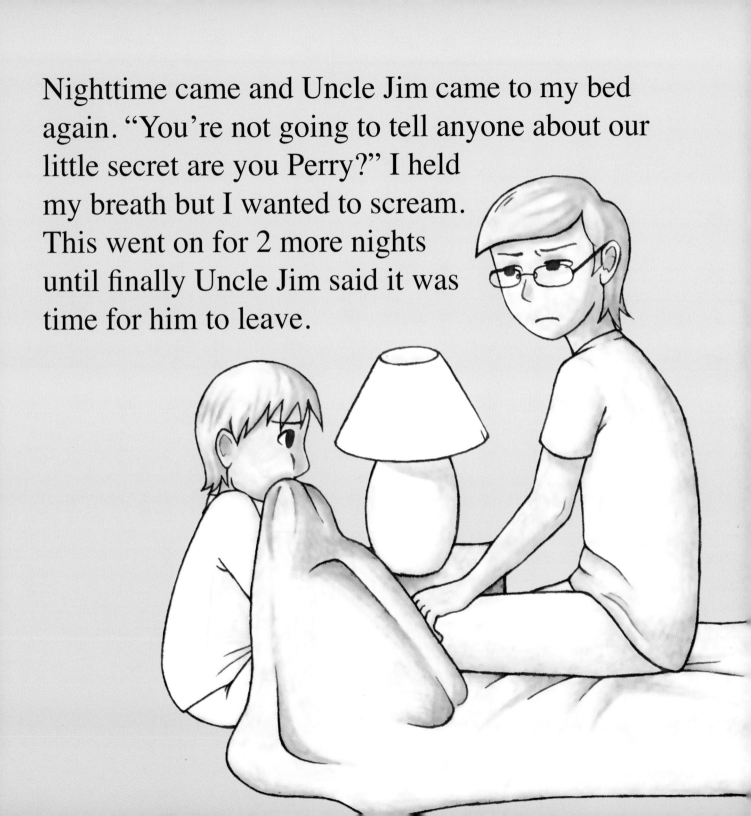

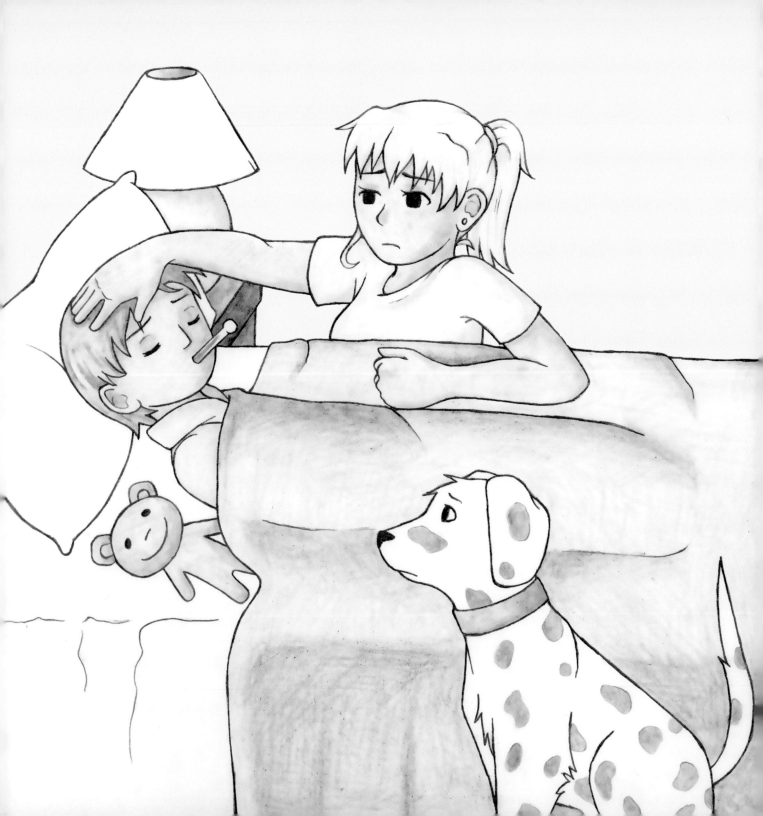

I stayed in bed for 2 more days
after he finally left. Mom said
I must have been under the
weather and that rest was the
best medicine. I finally got up
and dragged myself to school.
I wanted to tell someone about
Uncle Jim but I was afraid.
Would I get in trouble? What if
he came back to hurt me?

At school Mrs. Ash knew
something was not right. I got
in trouble 2 times for not paying
attention. Mrs. Ash pulled me
aside and asked me if there was
anything wrong. I told Mrs.
Ash about Uncle Jim. I tried
not to cry. She led
me straight to the
principals office
and made me
wait outside.
I was hoping I
wasn't in trouble.

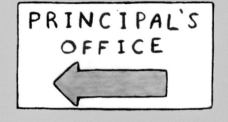

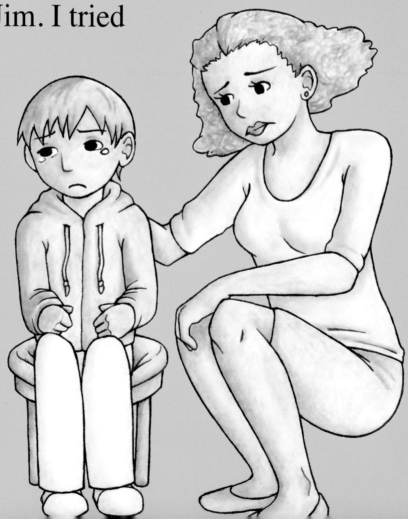

Mom and Dad came to the school quickly. Their eyes were wet and sad. Dad's face was red and Mom kept squeezing his arm. I sat with Mrs. Ash while Mom and Dad talked to the principal. After a while, Mom came out of the office and said it was time to go.

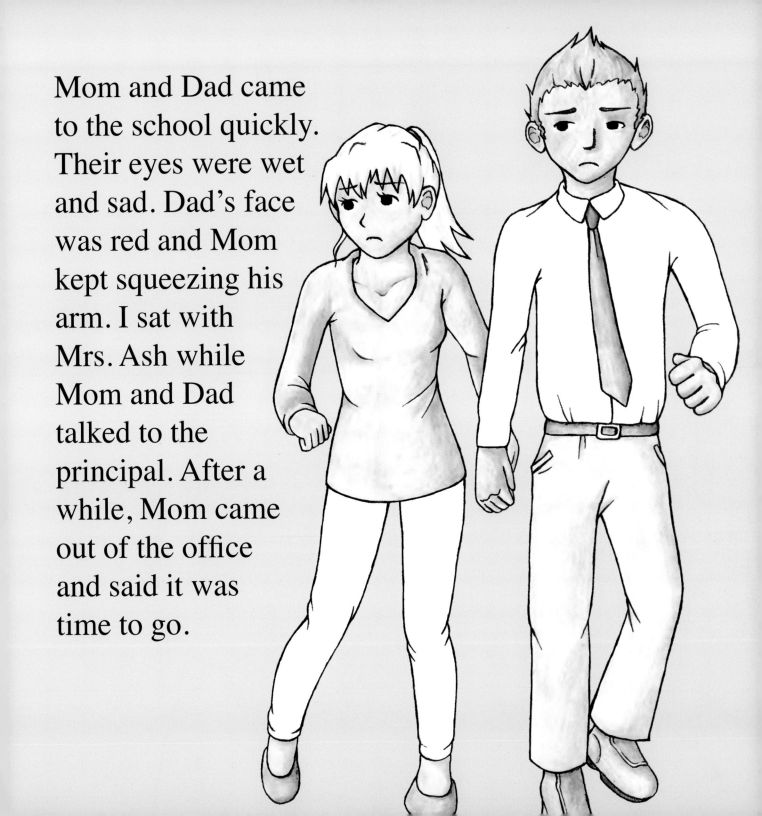

Dad said what happened to me wasn't my fault. He told me sometimes bad things happen like that it was good to tell someone like your teacher. He said I could always come to them or another trusted adult and tell the truth. He told me I wasn't in trouble and it didn't happen because I was bad. Mom couldn't bring herself to talk.

When we got home Mom made a phone call and about an hour later a policeman and a strange man called an investigator were ringing the doorbell. He wanted me to tell him what happened. I didn't want to tell but Mom said it was OK and to be brave.

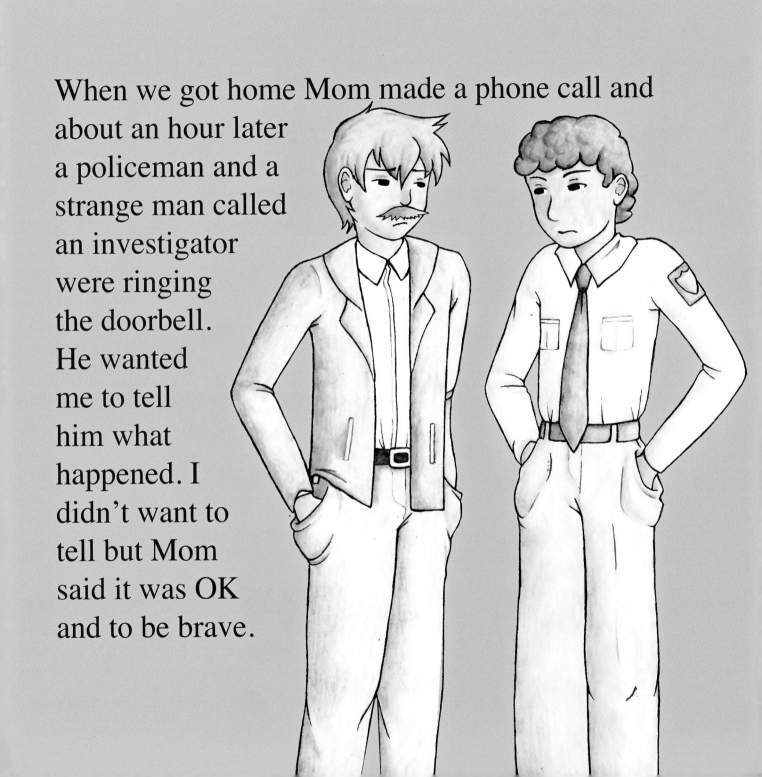

After they left Mom and Dad took me to the doctor. I don't like going to the doctor because I don't want a shot. Mom said Dr. Green would have to do an examination but they would be right there. Afterwards I got a sticker and a sucker.

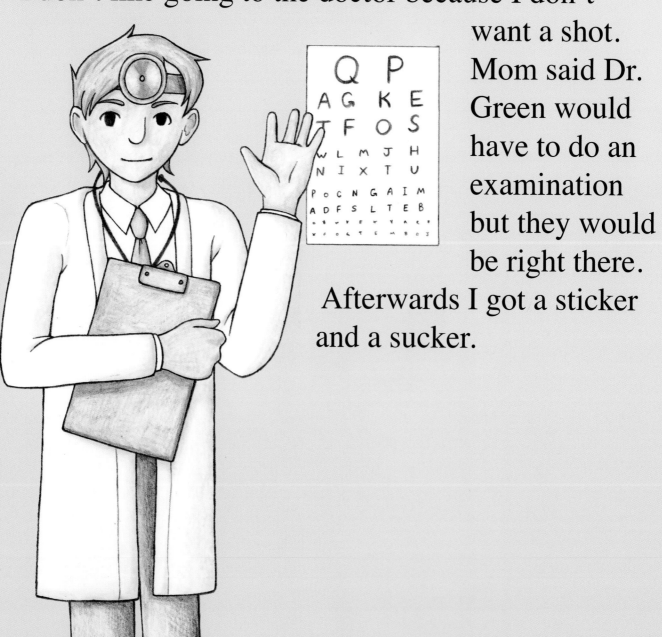

On the way home Dad said if someone tried to touch you or hurt you, you should tell your parents or a teacher. He said I didn't do anything wrong and that I did the right thing by telling Mrs. Ash.

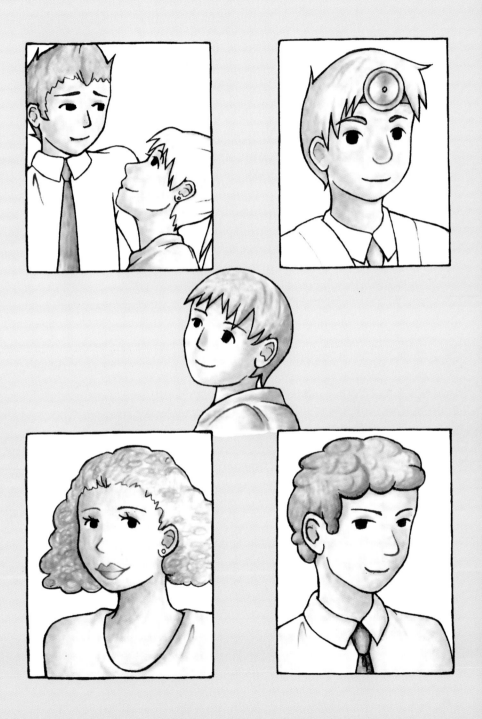

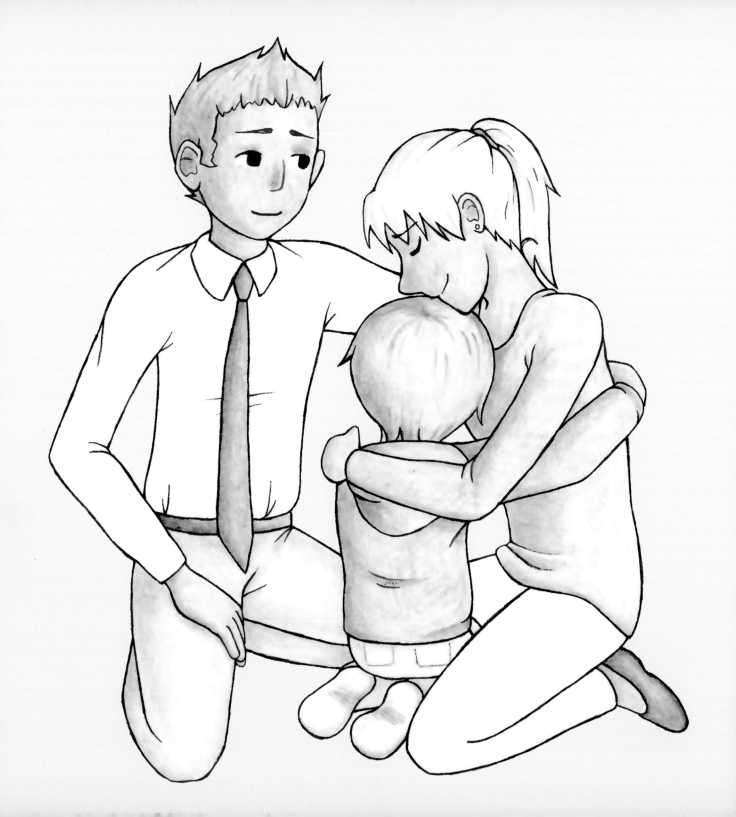

I now know it is not my fault.
I know that I am a good boy
and I know that I can trust
grown ups who care about me.
Mom said it is not good to
keep a secret like that and
that I did the right thing.

RESOURCES

Our Kids
1804 Haynes Street
Nashville, TN 37203
615-341-4911

Child Advocacy Center
1040 Samsonite Blvd
Murfreesboro, TN 37129
615-867-9000

Sexual Assault Center
101 French Landing Dr.
Nashville, TN 37228
615-259-9055

Boys and Girls Club
of Rutherford County
820 Jones Blvd
Murfreesboro, TN 37129
615-890-2582

United Way of Rutherford
and Cannon County
615 Memorial Blvd
Murfreesboro, TN 37129
615-893-7303